D0523495

if these BOOBS could talk

**a little humor
to pump up
the breastfeeding
mom**

T2-BVE-430

if these **BOOBS** could talk

a little humor to pump up
the breastfeeding mom

shannon payette seip & adrienne hedger

Andrews McMeel
Publishing, LLC

Kansas City

IF THESE BOOBS COULD TALK

Copyright © 2008 by Shannon Payette Seip and Adrienne Hedger. Illustrations copyright © 2008 by Adrienne Hedger. All rights reserved. Printed in Singapore. No part of this book may be used or reproduced in any manner whatsoever without written permission except in the case of reprints in the context of reviews. For information, write Andrews McMeel Publishing, LLC, an Andrews McMeel Universal company, 4520 Main Street, Kansas City, Missouri 64111.

08 09 10 11 12 TWP 10 9 8 7 6 5 4 3 2 1

ISBN-13: 978-0-7407-7120-0
ISBN-10: 0-7407-7120-5

Library of Congress Control Number: 2007934136

Book design by Diane Marsh

www.andrewsmcmeel.com

ATTENTION: SCHOOLS AND BUSINESSES
Andrews McMeel books are available at quantity discounts with bulk purchase for educational, business, or sales promotional use. For information, please write to: Special Sales Department, Andrews McMeel Publishing, LLC, 4520 Main Street, Kansas City, Missouri 64111.

BOOBS, this one's for you

When it comes to breastfeeding, people want to know: How is baby doing? Is she latching on? Is he eating well? How is baby's weight gain?

Baby this, baby that. Baby, baby, baby.

Well guess who starts to feel a wee bit slighted? That's right: your boobs. After all, *they* are the ones who are constantly delivering the goods. *They* are the ones who are negotiating tricky supply and demand issues. *They* are the ones who can't even recognize themselves in the mirror once the milk comes in.

But do they ever miss a day of work? No. Do they complain? Never. In fact, they are models of perseverance and flexibility. They are smart, fearless, and bodacious, all at once.

So, Boobs, for all that you do—and for all that you stand for—we dedicate this book to you.

v

SPECIAL DELIVERY!

Before you have a baby, it's only fair to warn your boobs about the changes ahead. Read them this letter before baby is born.

Dear Boobs,

How are you doing? Oh good.

Listen, life as you know it is about to end. There's a baby on the way, and this means big changes.

Let me put it this way: When normal people look at you they see breasts. When baby looks at you he sees something akin to a bucket of glistening, crispy chicken drumsticks. Mmmmm . . .

Suffice it to say, this baby will be attached to you for long periods of time, more frequently than you can imagine. And you will be called on to produce milk over and over and over again.

When times get tough, I want you to know I will be there to comfort you and cheer you on.

Maybe you already know all of this. After all, in many ways this assignment is your life's destiny. But in case you were unaware, I felt I should clue you in. I believe in you, and know you have what it takes to be the very best breasts.

I'll be seeing you (a LOT of you!) very soon. And don't worry—we'll get through this together.

Sincerely,
Me

top ten things your boobs would say if they could talk

1. Since when are we open twenty-four hours?

2. Get the soothing gel. Get it now.

3. Sir, this is a "Babies Only" zone.

4. Kid, how can you *not* see our nipples when they're the size of paper plates?

5. Woo hoo! We're spraying across the room!

6. Wow, we look spectacular!

7. Wait, now we look like old gym socks.

8. Hmmm, do we hear a baby crying somewh . . . and there's the milk.

9. Hey, we don't get paid enough to work this hard.

10. Oh great. A tooth.

REMIND ME: why am I going through all this?

Breastfeeding difficulties got you down? Take this quick quiz to remind yourself of the benefits you and your baby will enjoy.

1. Which answer is correct? When you breastfeed, your child has a lower risk of developing:
- a. A third nipple
- b. Respiratory problems
- c. An addiction to grande lattes
- d. A strong aversion to Barney—and his entire posse
- e. An attitude at age thirteen

2. True or false: When you breastfeed, your child has a greater chance of developing a higher IQ.

3. True or false: When you breastfeed, *you* have a greater chance of developing a higher IQ.

4. Breastfeeding can help you:
- a. Burn extra calories without having to hit the gym.
- b. Know your nipples intimately.
- c. Recover faster from postpartum bleeding.
- d. Make you look like a sex goddess in tank tops and low-cut shirts.
- e. All of the above.

ANSWERS:
Q1: B, although E would be great, too.
Q2: True! Yay!
Q3: Oh, please. Your brain is shot now that you won't be getting any sleep.
Q4: E, of course!

3

ENGORGED!

Your milk is here—and you can't believe what it feels like. Here's how to explain it to your spouse.

It's like:
- An alien replaced your boobs with fourteen-pound explosive bowling balls.
- Truck tires that are dangerously overinflated.
- A wicked witch cast a spell on you that makes your boobs as solid as stone.
- You're wearing a superhero chest-plate of steel, and the villain is shooting lasers at it.
- There's a miniature army in your boobs and they are punching you from the inside with their miniature fists.
- Your chest is the Hoover Dam and Lake Mead is pushing so hard, the dam is going to collapse in about two seconds.
- You went in to the hospital to give birth, but they accidentally gave you an enormous boob job.

If all this fails, relate it to him: It's like he woke up to find his testicles swollen to the size of grapefruits and as heavy as a pair of sandbags. (Oh yes, and burning like someone lit a bonfire inside of them.)

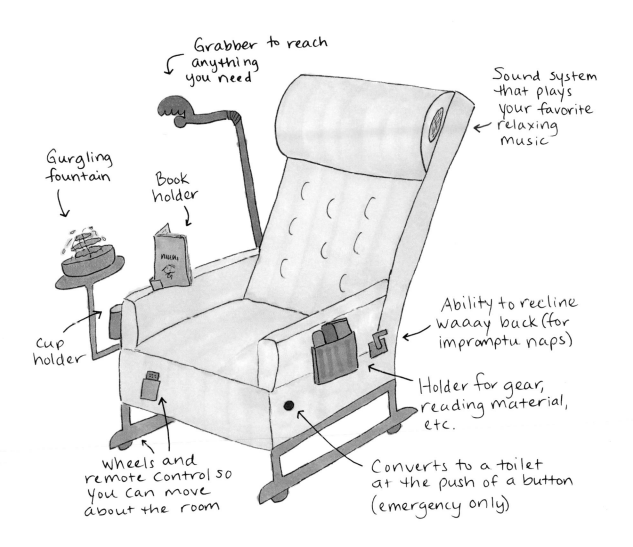

the **IDEAL ROCKER**

IS MY BABY LATCHED ON?

In the beginning, it can be difficult to determine if your baby has correctly latched to your breast. If you're in doubt, watch for these signs:

Good sign: Baby appears to be swallowing rhythmically.
Bad sign: Baby appears to be snoring rhythmically.

- -

Good sign: Your breast is decreasing in size somewhat. It is beginning to resemble an extremely overinflated football instead of a freakishly large watermelon.
Bad sign: After thirty minutes of supposed "feeding," your breasts are still so hard they could be registered as lethal weapons.

- -

Good sign: You feel a surge of milk rushing toward your nipple area.
Bad sign: You feel a surge of milk drenching your shirt, body, and baby.

- -

Good sign: There appears to be intense sucking going on.
Bad sign: The sensation of intense sucking is centered on your inner arm, where the baby's head is burrowed.

rock me, OXYTOCIN!

Wondering how to spend those fifteen seconds of breastfeeding you have *before* the oxytocin kicks in? Try the following:

- Recite the Pledge of Allegiance as if you were the world's most dramatic actor.
- Try tapping each toe, one by one, on the floor.
- Consider how you will manage the Tooth Fairy operation someday. How much money will you leave? What in the heck will you do with all those teeth?
- Try to recall exactly what you and your date wore to the prom—from your earrings to your date's matching cummerbund color.
- Using your tongue, count how many teeth you have.
- Try to spell your entire name backward.
- Give a motivational speech to your baby. Start by saying, "You're a winner, and I'm about to tell you why."
- Remember "Rock Me Amadeus" by Falco? Try singing this classic tune with the word "oxytocin" substituted for "Amadeus."
  Oxytocin! Oxytocin! Oh–Oh–Oh–Oxytocin!
  Rock me, Oxytocin!

top ten things that are worse than feeling like a dairy cow

Are you nursing so much you feel like a cow?
Life could be worse. Just be thankful you're not a:

1. Voodoo doll

2. Swollen blister on the verge of popping

3. Ugly piece of clothing that's been on
sale at 95 percent off for four years

4. Moldy, shriveled piece of fruit

5. Infected toenail that's cracked and yellowing

6. A $100 bill in Confederate money

7. Sun-warped cassette of Debbie Gibson, circa 1988

8. Pair of chopsticks being used by a three-year-old

9. Parking-meter enforcer

10. Can of Spam . . . that expired a year ago

BAD TIMES to BREASTFEED

#1: While competing in a bowling tournament

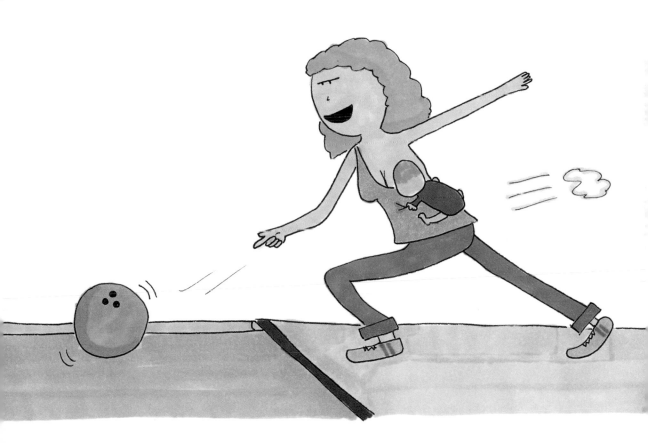

TRUE OR FALSE?

1. If baby falls asleep during nursing, you should do everything you can to wake her up and finish the feeding.
   Answer: True, but nearly impossible to accomplish.

2. The hunger cry is different from the tired cry.
   Answer: Supposedly true, but expect to go crazy as you try to figure it out.

3. A one-month-old baby typically takes in three ounces of milk in every feeding.
   Answer: True, but what good is this information when you are breastfeeding and have no idea if baby is ingesting one ounce or one gallon.

4. Sleep helps your body produce more milk.
   Answer: True. And what a cruel irony it is.

5. Breastfeeding helps you burn up to 500 calories per day.
   Answer: True. But sadly, that does not justify eating an entire pint of Ben & Jerry's Chocolate Fudge Brownie, which contains about 900 calories.

6. You cannot get pregnant while breastfeeding.
   Answer: False. Trust us. For the love of God, trust us.

YOU'RE WELCOME

Reasons your husband should be *thrilled* you are breastfeeding:

- It's FREE.
- He doesn't have to drag himself out of bed in the wee hours of the night to feed the baby—repeatedly.
- He also doesn't have to change baby's diaper in the middle of the night, then rechange it seconds later when baby poops in the clean diaper. Then repeat this scenario four more times.
- He can admire your spectacular pre-feeding session breasts—over and over again.
- Your child may have a higher IQ, which could lead to a better SAT score, which could lead to a full academic scholarship to college, which could spell early retirement for him.
- He isn't confronted with a sink full of bottles, nipples, and other feeding apparatus every time he walks into the kitchen.
- For the entire time you're breastfeeding, he doesn't have to concern himself *at all* with how, when, and where to feed the baby.

OUCH!

Believe it or not, there are some things that are worse than sore nipples. Consider these maladies:

- A paper cut on the eye
- Watching all seasons of *Saved by the Bell* in one sitting
- Finding gray hairs . . . way too many to pluck
- Sitting next to a gaseous passenger on an airplane
- Ordering takeout, getting home, and realizing you have the wrong order
- Getting stuck on the Whipper roller coaster
- Chewing the same piece of gum for an entire day
- Having your fingernail start to tear in a really, really low spot

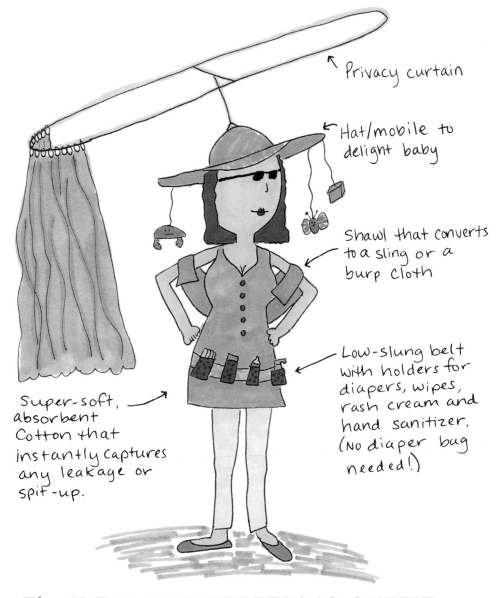

The **IDEAL BREASTFEEDING OUTFIT**

BOOB-TIONARY

Words that should be in the dictionary:

- **Lactidaisical**: aka "Baby Brain"
- **Bloppy**: The post-pregnancy fat that makes you feel like you're wearing a Boppy around your waist, even when you're not
- **Hengorgement**: The feeling that a dozen eggs have been planted under your boobs, making them rock hard and yet susceptible to splatting at any moment
- **Nip nap**: When you fall asleep nursing, exposing your nipple to the world
- **Breast plump**: The glory days when your waist is back to normal, but you still have lovely full boobs
- **Formulove**: When you switch to formula, and any guilt you feel is immediately replaced by a fierce love for this magical powder that transforms into something your baby will drink
- **Manolin**: When your husband uses your lanolin to cure his cracked heels
- **Ice age**: The era of pumping lots of milk to freeze so you can get a babysitter and go out
- **Nursing bla**: When you've just finished a long feeding and you catch a glimpse of your shrunken boobs . . . a preview of the shape of things to come when you finish nursing

PRESS ONE FOR BREAST MILK, PRESS TWO FOR . . .

Imagine if your boobs could produce other useful substances—besides milk. For instance:

Mace
So you could go out at night with no fear of attackers

Ketchup
For those times you go through the drive-through but it's too messy to open ketchup packets for your fries

Sunscreen and bug spray
In case you forgot them at home and are headed to the park

Gasoline
With gas prices sky high, you'd be able to afford a shopping spree

Antibacterial hand gel
When there's not a sink around after you change a dirty diaper

Saline
When dirt gets trapped on your contact, you can take it out, squirt it with some boob saline, and pop it back in

Infant gas drops
Top off a big feeding by switching to "Infant Gas Drop" mode. Sound sleep ahead!

WD-40
Rocker starting to squeak? Nursery doorknob a bit sticky? Problem solved.

GET TO YOUR HUNGRY BABY

Oops! It's feeding time and you're out of the house.
Can you find your way back to baby?

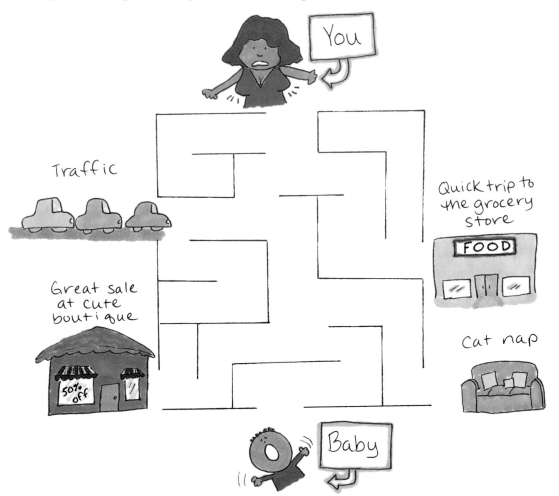

WHAT TO DO if you're leaking with no baby in sight

Have your boobs sprung a leak at an inconvenient time? These tips will help you make the best of an awkward situation:

- Hum or sing the theme to *Titanic*.
- If you are holding a beverage, subtly pour it on your shirt so you're wet all over and everything blends in. (Note: Do not use a hot beverage; that will cause other problems.)
- Be productive—discreetly use your breast milk to water the nearest wilted plant.
- Look for a fire to put out, preferably a small fire.
- Start panting and wiping your forehead to create the illusion you just finished a five-mile run and the leaking is actually chest sweat (more believable if you are not wearing a skirt and heels).
- Make a beeline for the nearest bowl of cereal—it's perfectly good milk, after all.
- Embrace the beauty of the moment. Strike a pose (preferably on a sloping lawn) in the position of a beautiful fountain with water shooting from your nipples.
- If your milk starts to pour out with fire-hoselike intensity, try to remove paint chips or stubborn debris on your house. At this point, it's all about multitasking.

WHAT'S IN A NAME?

Since there's so much attention paid to your breasts, surely they deserve their own names. Take this quiz to find out which names fit your boobs best!

1. Yippee! You've just found a babysitter for Saturday. What's your ideal way to spend your few free hours?
   a. Rock climbing
   b. Comedy club
   c. A night out with some girlfriends
   d. Shopping
   e. Going for a bike ride

2. Which of the following was the biggest reason you got in trouble as a child?
   a. Stealing the car
   b. Playing practical jokes
   c. Talking too long on the telephone
   d. Whining
   e. Beating up on your sibling

3. At a carnival, which of the following do you head to first?
   a. Tilt-a-whirl
   b. Fun house
   c. Ferris wheel
   d. You would never be seen at a carnival
   e. Bell-and-hammer game (hit the hammer, ring the bell)

4. If you were going to rent a movie, it would most likely be:
   a. *The Wizard of Oz*
   b. *Meet the Parents*
   c. *Beaches*
   d. *Pretty Woman*
   e. *GI Jane*

WHAT'S IN A NAME? answer key

If you answered mostly:

· ·

As

You should name your boobs:

THELMA and LOUISE

You're the daring type who's always up for an adventure!

Bs

You should name your boobs:

LUCY and ETHEL

You've got a silly bone that gets groups giggling!

Cs

You should name your boobs:

RACHEL and MONICA

You're a devoted friend and adore your bosom buddies!

Ds

You should name your boobs:

MARY KATE and ASHLEY

You've got it all and have no time to waste on the little people.

Es

You should name your boobs:

SERENA and VENUS

You're a star athlete and a wonder woman!

20

Y ou . . .

- Have no qualms going to your niece's graduation with spit-up all over your dress
- Let your toddler practice face painting on not just your face but both of your boobs while your baby is nursing
- Would rather pee next to the playground in plain sight than schlep all the baby stuff—and your kid—to the nearest restroom two blocks away
- Don't flinch when changing a poopy diaper on the floor of your accountant's office during a meeting
- Don't mind going to your husband's work party without taking a shower . . . for the past three days
- Recount your graphic birth story for all the relatives at a family reunion

THAT'S the NAME?

Do your relatives question the name you selected for your baby? Just point out that it could have been worse: You could have selected a truly "unique" name, following the tradition of Hollywood celebrities.

What name might you choose if you were a famous actor? To figure it out, use this simple formula:

The name = the third item on your grocery list

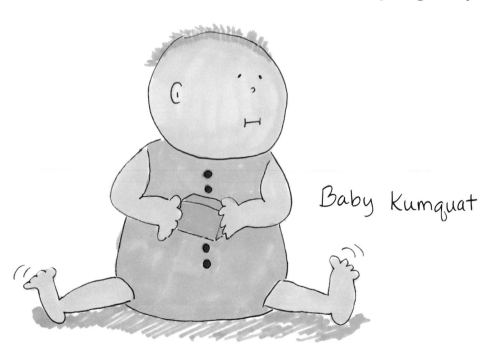

Baby Kumquat

TAKING SIDES

Did you misplace that little safety pin that reminds you which breast is first at the next feeding? Don't fret! Try these alternate approaches to keep track of what side you should start on:

- Tilt your head to the proper side and hold it there until the next feeding.
- Apply lipstick to only that side of your lips.
- Walk with that foot first.
- Only turn that direction in your car.
- Wear a soccer shin guard on the appropriate leg.
- Switch the part of your hair.
- Pop the lens out of that side of your glasses.
- Write only with that hand.
- Refer to yourself as Lucy (for left) or Regina (for right).
- Apply fake eyelashes to that eye.
- Respond to everyone by saying either "Right-O," or "Let loose."

BAD TIMES to BREASTFEED

#2: While learning to in-line skate

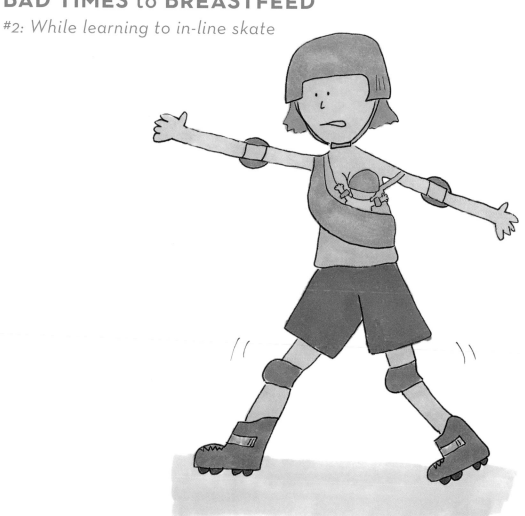

ONCE UPON A FEEDING

Use the guidelines below to select a list of words. Then fill in the blanks to the right to create your own personalized story!

_____
Adjective

_____
Adjective that is an emotion

_____
Adjective

_____
An article of clothing or an accessory

_____
Verb ending in "ing"

_____
Plural noun

_____
Number

_____
Line from a song

_____
Adjective

_____
Number

24

From the get-go, I knew it would be a _____ nursing session.
(adjective)

The baby was in a _____ mood and was inexplicably wearing
(adjective-emotion)

a _____ _____ . I had just finished _____ with a
(adjective) (clothing) (verb-ing)

couple _____ . But it had been _____ minutes since
(plural noun) (number)

baby's last meal, so it was definitely time to eat! We settled in, and

25

as baby looked up at me I lovingly said, "_____ ." Soon after, I
(line from song)

noticed baby was sound asleep. Feeling exhausted and _____ ,
(adjective)

I closed my eyes as well. We rested for _____ minutes—the
(number)

longest I've slept in months.

FACE THE FACTS

Match the face to the situation.

- Your husband wants to get intimate.

- Your nipple is bleeding—again.

- It's been several hours, and you need to feed someone NOW.

- You just laid down for a quick nap and your baby started crying again.

- You just realized you forgot to return your friend's urgent phone call . . . from ten days ago.

- You're trying to assemble your super-duper, ultrapowerful pump for the first time.

- You're trying to remember when you last showered.

- You just remembered you still have twelve thank-you notes to write for new-baby gifts.

- Your visitors are forty-five minutes late, completely throwing off the feeding schedule you painstakingly arranged specifically for this visit.

it's time to BORST-feed!

Are you getting tired of hearing the word breast?
Try these translations on for size:

Spanish = *pecho*
Chinese = *rufang*
Indonesian = *buah dada*
German = *brust*
Hebrew = *chazeh*
Italian = *seno*
Swahili = *kifua*
Portuguese = *pieto*
Dutch = *borst*
Afrikaans = *bors*
Vietnamese = *thú lỗi*
Albanian = *gji*
Finnish = *rinta*
Romanian = *piept*
Swedish = *bröst*
Pig Latin = *eastbray*

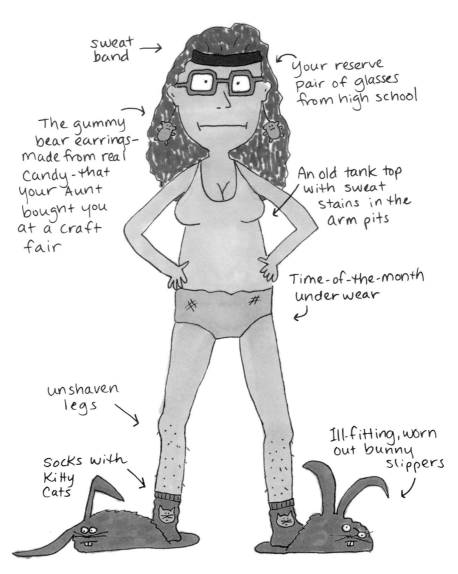

WHAT'S LESS SEXY THAN A NURSING BRA?

THE NAME GAME

You might feel like an extra on *ER* because you've heard so many words that have to do with breastfeeding. Can you match the word to its correct meaning? (See answers on the next page.)

Meanings

1. Rooting reflex

a. Anything that excites lactation. Such as the cry of a random baby who is a mile away.

2. Hoffman maneuver

b. Seed that is said to help enrich breast milk. (Also sounds like the name of that weird guy who lived down the street from you in college.)

3. Fenugreek

c. Breast pain. Doctors may choose to say this more complicated word. You may choose to say AAAAAHHHHHHHHHHHH!!!!

4. Galactagogue

d. When baby turns his face toward your boob and makes sucking motions. Particularly amusing when baby does this to strangers.

5. Mammalgia

6. Oxytocin

e. Cream applied to sore, cracked nipples. It may soon mean more to you than your very own siblings.

7. Lanolin

f. The hormone responsible for the let-down reflex. (Ahhhh . . . It doesn't get better than this.)

8. Colostrum

g. What your boobs produce before your milk comes in. Sort of like a newborn's appetizer.

h. Method of erecting nipples to help feed baby. (The very act that may have landed you into motherhood.)

THE NAME GAME answers

1. **d ROOTING REFLEX**—When baby turns his face toward your boob and makes sucking motions

2. **h HOFFMAN MANEUVER**—Method of erecting nipples to help feed baby

3. **b FENUGREEK**—Seed said to help enrich breast milk. (No, not that weird guy down the street.)

4. **a GALACTAGOGUE**—Anything that excites lactation

5. **c MAMMALGIA**—Breast pain (aka AAAAAHHHHHHHHHHHH!!!!)

6. **f OXYTOCIN**—Hormone responsible for the let-down reflex

7. **e LANOLIN**—Cream applied to sore, cracked nipples

8. **g COLOSTRUM**—The "newborn appetizer"

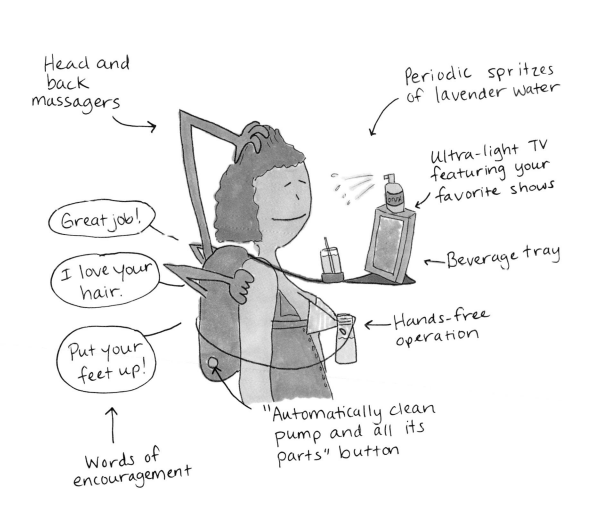

The **IDEAL BREAST PUMP**

HOW TO encourage your baby to take a bottle

Is baby having trouble adjusting to a bottle? You're not alone. But you may find success with this tried and true ten-step method:

1. Dim the lights.

2. Turn on soothing music.

3. Snuggle up to baby.

4. Softly say, "Here comes the little bottle."

5. Gently touch bottle nipple to baby's lower lip.

6. Watch as baby's face scrunches into horrified expression.

7. Flinch as baby violently swats bottle to the floor.

8. Sigh a deep sigh.

9. Bend down and pick up bottle.

10. Begin at step one again. Repeat roughly 1,192 times, until one day—for no particular reason whatsoever—baby decides to accept bottle.

now that's a WORKOUT!

Breastfeeding can burn up to 500 calories per day. So while you sit calmly nursing your baby, you burn the same number of calories you would if you completed:

- One hour of high-impact aerobics
- One hour of mowing the lawn with a push mower
- One hour of shoveling snow
- One hour of chopping and splitting wood
- One hour of coal mining
- One hour of horse grooming
- Ninety minutes of hunting
- More than ninety minutes of hunching over and bathing a dog
- Two hours of paddle-boating
- Two hours of mopping
- Two and a half hours of applying fertilizer to your lawn
- Three hours of brushing your teeth
- Five hours of standing in a line
- Seven hours of making out with your spouse

top ten most surprising
things about breastfeeding

1. How many holes there are when the milk comes out of your nipple

2. How much they deflate after a feeding

3. How quickly they fill back up

4. How many days in a row you can wear your
favorite nursing bra

5. How fast and easy it is to prepare your baby's meal

6. How satisfying it is to coax a little burp from your baby

7. How absolutely thirsty you get while nursing

8. How it can take almost an hour for baby to eat
an entire meal of three ounces

9. How your baby can just fall right asleep,
smack in the middle of a meal

10. How a person can enjoy eating the same thing,
every meal, every day for months on end

BOOBS AT A PLAYDATE

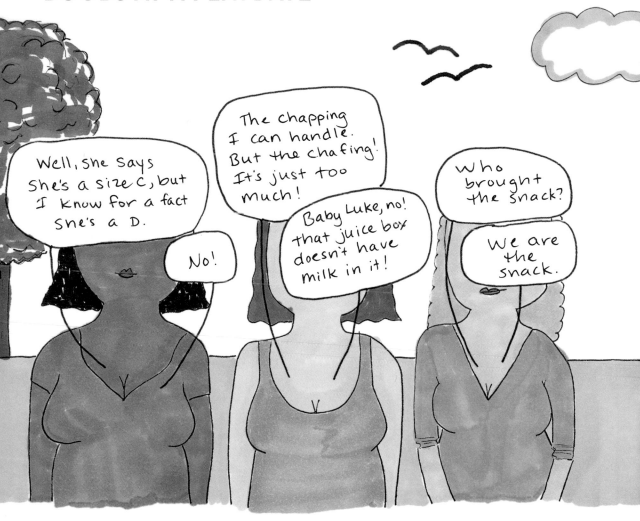

HOW TO motivate your boobs to produce more milk

- Create an inspiring soundtrack with songs like "Eye of the Tiger."

- Enroll them in a Tony Robbins course.

- Create a sticker reward chart.

- Refuse to have sex with your husband until your boobs cooperate.

- Increase their circle of influence, and introduce them to friends' boobs who are extremely productive.

- Hang posters that say things like "Attitudes are contagious. Is yours worth catching?"*

- Live near a dairy farm? Visit the dairy cows and let your boobs watch the masters at work.

*See poster on page 87 to give your boobs a motivational lift.

HOW TO reward your boobs when they do produce more milk

- Present them with a gift certificate for a day at the spa (or just a soak in your tub—they won't be able to tell the difference).

- Let them have control of the remote for the evening.

- Surprise them with a box of truffles, or any other delicacy that has some resemblance to boobs.

- Sew them a new couture pair of nursing pads.

- Let them roam free in your tank top—no nursing bra—for the entire morning.

- Purchase tasteful jewelry for them (avoid sharp points and pierced items, so as not to harm them).

who HASN'T seen your boobs?

Let's face it: When your boobs become a food source, your personal privacy takes a hit. Just how exposed are you? Take a look at this list and put a check mark next to each person or group of people who has NOT seen one of your boobs.

O Your baby (hopefully you don't check this one)

O Your husband (hopefully you don't check this one)

O Your entire playgroup

O A large dog

O A small dog

O A waitress serving pancakes

O Your father-in-law

- Your neighbor's goldfish

- The women's restroom attendant at Nordstrom

- The UPS driver

- The UPS driver's stand-in

- Your pastor

- Any member of the circus

- A group of seniors riding a tour bus

- Your state senator

- A class of second-graders

- Your cousin's girlfriend's roommate—and her friend

- The stranger squeezed in next to you on the plane

- Every parent in your toddler's playgroup

- The staff at the Picture People photo store at the mall

- An Elvis impersonator

- The guy who plays the saxophone on the street corner

- Everyone who ate lunch at Arby's at 12:45 p.m. last Thursday

ANSWERS
If you checked:

0-5 boxes
Britney Spears? Paris Hilton? They've got nothing on the amount of exposure your boobs have seen.

6-10 boxes
Your boobs are very social and have several admirers. You must be proud!

10 or more boxes
While you are incredibly modest, your boobs are yearning to see more sunlight.

TYPES OF HOLDS YOU DON'T FIND IN BOOKS

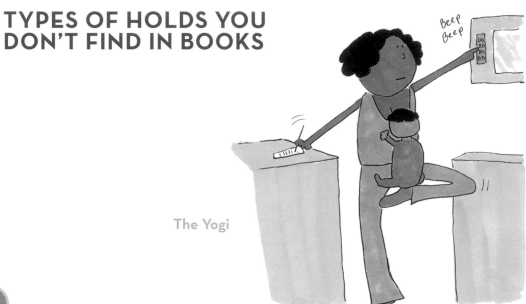

The Yogi

The Techie

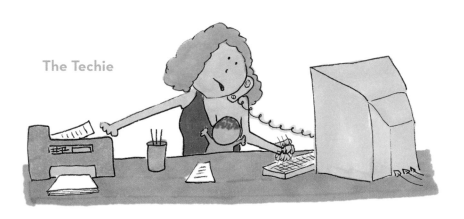

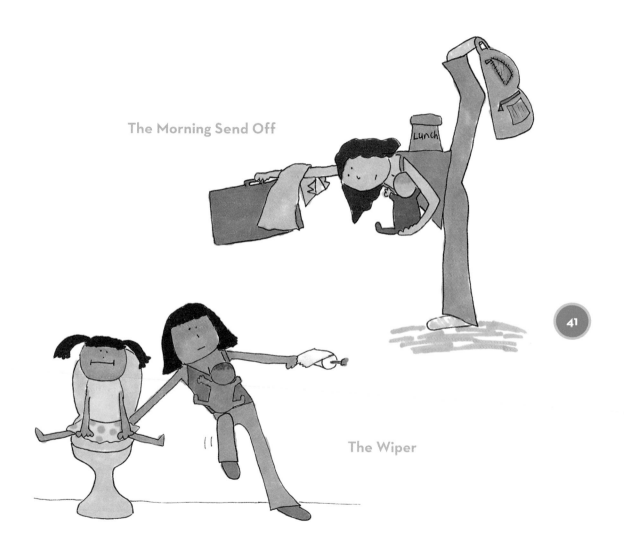

The Morning Send Off

The Wiper

41

EXPERT ADVICE FROM A BREAST

Dear Breast,

Why does it sometimes take a long time for the milk to let down?

—Waiting for Milkman

Dear "Waiting,"

Well gee. I'd like to see you try to deal with breast tissue, alveoli, the lactiferous sinuses, milk fat globules, and milk ducts—not to mention continual interruptions from the central nervous system—in just a matter of seconds. Truly, it's a wonder that we breasts are even able to produce milk. Why don't you consider that as you wait—patiently, I might add— for the milk to come.

—Breast

Dear Breast,

I feel like my breasts have a mind of their own. We used to be close, but now I hardly even recognize them.

—Missing the Twins

Dear "Missing the Twins,"

Imagine that you wake up one morning to find that you are expected to run twenty marathons in a row . . . starting now! No training, no experience! Just go! Would you be concerned about communicating with others, or would you just be focused on the overwhelming task at hand? Your breasts are now marathon runners. Let them be.

—Breast

HOW TO console a rejected breast

Occasionally, babies will shun one breast in favor of the other. It's not only hard on you; it's difficult for the rejected breast. Consider these coping strategies:

- Don't let the rejected breast get depressed. Reassure your breast; let it know that it is still a critical part of your body. Perhaps sing it a Celine Dion song.
- Explain to your infant that, despite any underutilization, milk continues to aggregate in the clusters of alveoli and the milk ducts in your breast, creating an inconvenient situation for you. Getting a blank stare in return? Explain again, this time slower and with more enunciation.
- Use face paint to decorate the rejected breast as a bunny or fanciful woodland creature. This may engage baby's interest. Do not create any sort of ominous appearance, or you will risk deeper trouble.
- Invite your rejected breast and your baby to the same place at the same time. (Don't tell them that the other will be there). This "chance encounter" could help them fall in love all over again.

FIND YOUR BED

It's 2:00 a.m. and you just finished feeding baby.
Can you find your way back to bed?

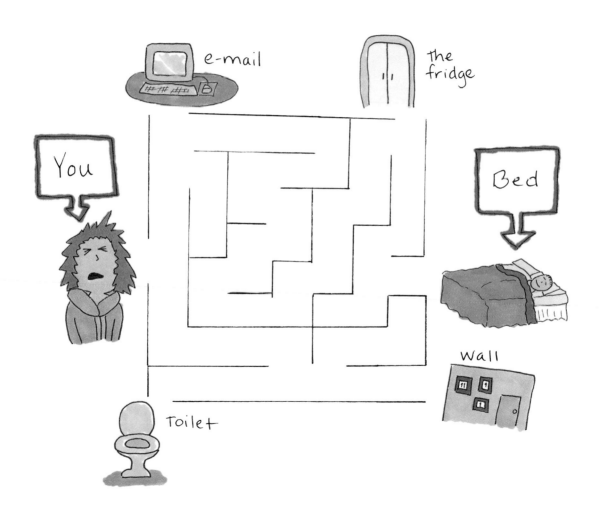

top ten breast-friendly cities in the united states

1. Mollie's Nipple, California

2. Nipple Mountain, Colorado

3. Two Tits, California

4. Nip, Missouri

5. The Nipples, Arizona

6. Two Teats, California

7. Feeding Hills, Massachusetts

8. Nellie's Nipple, California

9. Sucker Flat, California

10. Short Pump, Virginia

things your husband did
NOT EVER WANT TO KNOW,
OK?!! JEEZ!

- Your milk ducts can become clogged, requiring you to squeeze a mucous plug out of your nipple.

- Your breast can squirt milk across the entire room.

- You can get a yeast infection on your breasts.

- You've been fitted for nipple shields.

- Your breast milk may have a green or yellow tint.

- That your boobs will never be this big again, and NO, he cannot fondle them.

- If he does fondle them, he may get a milk bath.

HOROSCOPE FOR BREASTFEEDING BOOBS

Find your boobs' sign (hint: same as your sign), then read them their horoscope so they know what to expect in the coming days.

. . . .

Aries (March 21–April 19)
You struggle with feelings of jealousy over friends who seem to have more spare time.

Taurus (April 20–May 20)
Your goals will come to fruition. Keep your eyes on the prize—thirty ounces a day.

Gemini (May 21–June 21)
Be prepared for an unfortunate surprise, like baby throw-up splattered all over you. Fortunately, you will soon forget this incident.

Cancer (June 22–July 22)
A new bra will soon be your neighbor and your friend. You will bring out the best in each other.

Leo (July 23–August 22)
There's a little someone who can't keep his eyes off you. It's going to be a busy day.

Virgo (August 23–September 22)
Break out of your comfort zone, and try something new.
Perhaps a non-nursing bra (just for a few hours!).

Libra (September 23–October 23)
Tensions arise between the two of you. Get to the root
of it. Explore the roots of your angst and apologize for
past wrongdoings.

Scorpio (October 24–November 21)
Don't hide behind those nipple shields any longer. It's time
to introduce the world to the real you.

Sagittarius (November 22–December 21)
Let go of your hatred of pureed vegetables. Baby was bound
to eat them eventually. It's not your fault.

Capricorn (December 22–January 19)
Obstacles are headed your way, particularly in the form of teeth.

Aquarius (January 20–February 18)
Demand will outpace supply over the next three days. Get ready
for more production.

Pisces (February 19–March 20)
You will feel drained and empty. The source of this issue will
turn out to be a tiny human with a big appetite.

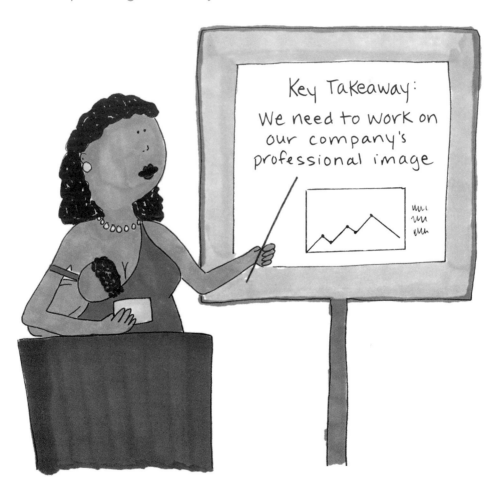

GIVE AND TAKE

Things you do for your baby that you hope he _never_ has to do for you:
- Administer a suppository
- Breastfeed
- Rub on yeast infection cream
- Assist with circumcision
- Remove accidental poop from bathtub
- Peel off clothing in the middle of the store
- Use booger snatcher to suck out mucus
- Give a time-out

Things you do for your baby that you hope he _will_ do for you:
- Pay for new clothes every few months
- Sweep floor at least once a day
- Give hugs and kisses
- Bribe with treats
- Rub back every night
- Drive you everywhere you need to go
- Encourage you to take a nap

WHAT HAPPENED TO BABY?

Put on your detective hat and try to figure out what happened to baby.

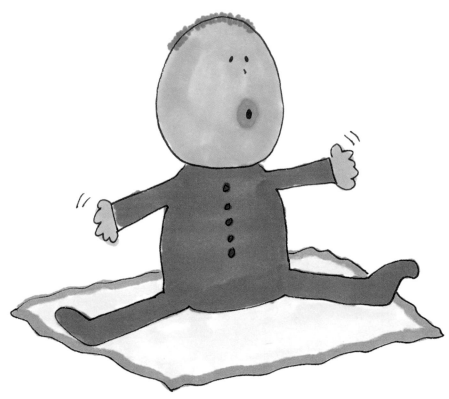

ANSWER:
Oops! You breastfed baby right after you applied your self tanner.

the top ten things you can do
when you're up for a 2:15 a.m. feeding
and can't fall back asleep

1. Practice different accents without anyone laughing.

2. Spin a 1980s tune and see if you can still bust a move.

3. Rummage through your stash of beauty products and see if you can unearth ten that you haven't touched in a year.

4. Eat an entire pint of Häagen-Dazs ice cream, then lick the bowl sparkling clean.

5. Watch reruns of the shows you really like, but would never admit in public (*Jerry Springer, ALF, Baywatch*).

6. See if you can squeeze your way into your pre-pregnancy jeans.

7. Go outside and lie down in the doghouse, just for a change of pace and company.

8. Practice the moonwalk.

9. Pretend you could pause time, then imagine all the ways you would use this power tomorrow.

10. Create three to four giant, nonhuman footprints in a nearby patch of grass and see if any neighbors freak out in the morning.

THEN AND NOW

WHAT YOU THOUGHT ABOUT BEFORE BABY	WHAT YOU THINK ABOUT NOW
Work	Planning everything you need to pack in the car and diaper bag to take a short drive to the grocery store
Date nights	Poop, pee, how much, when, where
A great novel	Chapter 7 of *How to Get Your Baby to Sleep Through the Night*
Talking to your friend about the season finale of your favorite show	Talking to your friend about mastitis
Traveling to the Caribbean	Traveling to the nearest pediatrician's office
Which outfit to wear to an upcoming social event	Which outfit has any hope of still fitting
Sex = fun	Sex = another item on the to-do list. And unfortunately it's not ranking too high.

DOODLE TOES

Using a pencil between your toes while breastfeeding or pumping, draw a portrait of what you think your child will look like in ten years.

(Now hope like the dickens you're wrong.)

Did you know?

1. Norway is the only country to include breast milk in national food statistics.

2. The Philippines earned a unique *Guinness Book of World Records* achievement when 3,738 mothers nursed their babies simultaneously in Manila.

3. A study published in the June 2004 issue of the *New England Journal of Medicine* shows that breast milk is known to cure warts.

4. If moms got paid minimum wage for working *twenty hours* a day, *seven* days a week (assuming they're getting four hours of sleep a night), they'd make $37,492 each.

5. Kangaroos sometimes nurse their young until they're the same size as the mothers. Yikes!

HOW TO HANDLE A NURSING STRIKE

1. Call all parties to the table. (A low coffee table works best since you may need to prop baby up with a pillow.)

2. Explain that you understand a strike is under way and you are open to negotiation.

3. Ask your baby to state the root cause of the strike. (Does he want a softer blanket? A more entertaining mobile? A stylish little hat?)

4. Wait for your baby to respond with any type of noise. Do not rush in to fill the silence, just wait. (Good negotiators don't mind silence; often the opposing party will get anxious and quickly compromise.)

5. Once baby makes a noise, try to discern its meaning. Is he truly cooperating with this negotiation or did he just poop his pants?

6. Either way, switch to Plan B: Explain to baby that if he nurses—even just a tiny bit—you are prepared to write him a check for $100,000, on the spot.

7. If this tactic is met with silence, implement Plan C: a dab of vanilla ice cream on your nipple.

8. If baby is intrigued by this turn of events, pat yourself on the back. Realize the negotiations with this pint-sized human will get ten times harder every year. There will be fewer and fewer issues that can be solved with a dab of ice cream on your breast.

WAYS TO MULTITASK WHILE BREASTFEEDING

DEFROST PEAS
Effort level:
*20% (open and
close freezer)*

Payoff:
*Depends on how
much you like peas*

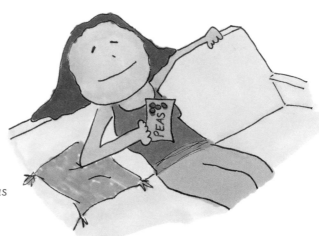

APPLY MAKEUP
Effort level:
*0% (you)
30% (baby)*

Payoff:
*The longer she eats,
the better you look*

WORK OUT
Effort level:
100%

Payoff:
Burn the breastfeeding calories, plus some!

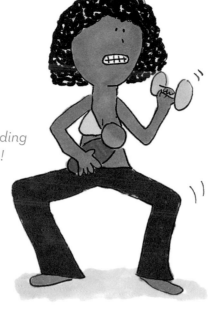

SLEEP
Effort level:
0%

Payoff:
Pure Bliss

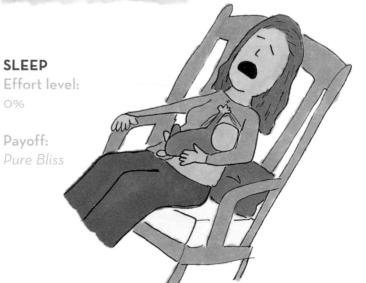

A MORNING IN THE LIFE OF
A BREASTFEEDING MOM

5:30 a.m.
Awake and drag yourself out of bed, off couch, or up from floor to attend to wailing baby.

5:32 a.m.
Grab huge glass of ice water. Get comfortable. Begin feeding baby.

5:36 a.m.
Look down to find baby is asleep on your boob. Appreciate irony that you would give anything—*anything!*—for twenty minutes of sleep. Yet here you are trying to wake someone else up.

5:37 a.m.
Wake baby so boobs don't explode.

5:40 a.m.
Continue feeding baby. Realize you are now sitting in an awkward, hunched-over position. Decide to remain put (best not to disturb baby).

5:41–5:44 a.m.
Guzzle entire glass of ice water (as you continue to breastfeed in an awkward, hunched-over position).

5:45 a.m.
Realize you need to go to the bathroom—immediately.

5:48 a.m.
Stop breastfeeding and lay baby on blanket. Dash to the bathroom. Hear baby's cry and experience crushing guilt every second that you are peeing. Sprint back to baby; resume breastfeeding.

5:55 a.m.
Realize you could really use your inflatable donut, since your hemorrhoids are acting up.

5:56 a.m.
Realize that the last thing in the world you feel like doing is hunting down your inflatable donut.

6:00 a.m.
Look down to see that baby is asleep once again.

6:01 a.m.
Surrender. Lay your head back and get some shut-eye yourself, knowing you'll repeat the schedule in a matter of minutes.

HOW TO FIND YOUR INNER HOTTIE

Sure, you may feel frumpy, but use your imagination—and the chart below—to reenvision yourself as *fabulous*!

WHAT THE WORLD SEES	WHAT YOU PICTURE IN YOUR HEAD
Minivan	Audi convertible
Stretch marks	Belly button ring
Diaper bag	Kate Spade purse
Extra cellulite	Airbrushed, perfectly tan legs
Nursing bra	Victoria's Secret Very Sexy bra
Baby Einstein	"She's My Cherry Pie" by Warrant
Baggy eyes	Fresh-from-the-spa glow
Rocking chair	Bar stool at hip, celebrity-filled L.A. club
What to Expect Baby's First Year	Latest issue of *Vogue*

BAD TIMES to BREASTFEED

#4: During acupuncture therapy

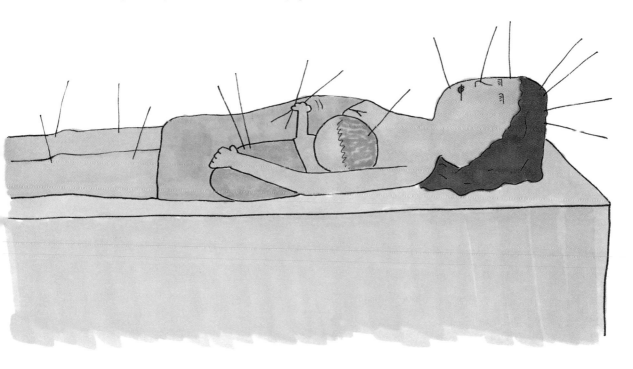

would you RATHER . . . ?

- Be forced to create a diaper using only uncooked lasagna noodles and Scotch tape, or play peekaboo for six hours straight?

- Eat a pureed onion for lunch every day or be swaddled tightly before going to bed each night?

- Continue wearing only your maternity clothes for the next year or be forced to get rid of all of your maternity/transition clothes right this second?

- Have absolutely no information about the first year's developmental milestones or receive a phone call updating you with information every hour?

- Pour out all your stored breast milk or parade down the beach in a thong bikini?

HOW WILL YOU waste the most
money in the early months of motherhood?

- Buying every single brand of bottle and nipple on the market, none of which your baby will accept

- Buying clothes a size too big, then a size too small, then clothes that actually fit but are totally inconvenient for breastfeeding

- Buying the extra-jumbo pack of size 1 diapers, then realizing that your baby is now a solid size 2

- Enrolling your baby in several classes, only to learn that your little one wants *out* of the pool during swimming lessons, sleeps during music class, and wails during baby yoga

- Buying your baby a ton of adorable clothes, but stuffing the closet so full that she never wears half of them because you can't actually see anything in the closet

- Purchasing three different strollers, two swings (one for upstairs and downstairs), an ExerSaucer, a bouncy chair, and two backpacks (one for you and your hubby), then discovering you don't have time or energy to assemble any of it

- Going on a major shopping spree when you get back to your pre-pregnancy weight, only to realize that your body is *still* morphing

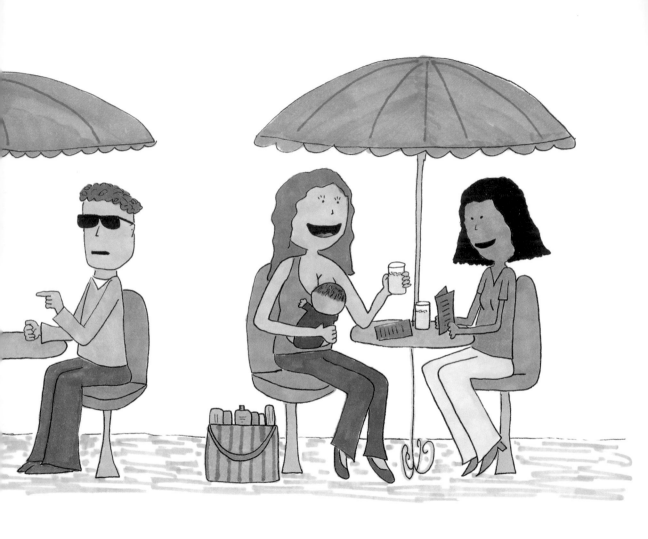

WHAT'S WRONG WITH THIS PICTURE?

WHAT'S WRONG
WITH THIS PICTURE? answers

- Hair and makeup done? Puh-leez.

- Baby isn't distracted and/or pulling mom's shirt down to display her boob to the world.

- No one is gawking at the breastfeeding mom.

- That diaper bag is *way* too neat.

- Wait: are those pre-maternity jeans?? Did she even *have* a baby?

- Water? I don't think so. Mom wouldn't look that alert without a little caffeine.

WORD SCRAMBLE

Can you figure out what breastfeeding-related words appear below?

tnalaocit uoctntasln

_____ _____

gusnirn apd

_____ _____

stbaer mppu

_____ _____

enlpip dheisl

_____ _____

issmtati

_____

hhrtsu

_____

al elehc ualeeg

_____ _____ _____

usoocltmr

_____

ANSWERS:
Lactation consultant
Nursing pad
Breast pump
Nipple shield
Mastitis
Thrush
La Leche League
Colostrum

YOUR BREASTS' SUPERPOWERS

- Can instantly silence a screaming infant

- Able to triple their size in just one night

- Will easily shoot milk across a room, stunning onlookers

- Are activated by even the faintest baby cry

- Unassumingly contain all the food a little human needs for several months

- Can reduce you to tears or fill you with joy—sometimes both at the same time

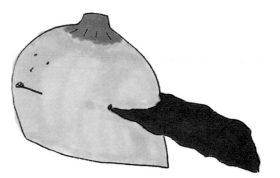

GUILT TRIP vs. REALITY

A h, breastfeeding. There's the bonding . . . the wondrous moments . . . the endless guilt trips.

GUILT TRIP YOU PULL ON YOURSELF	REALITY
My baby is crying. Yes, she just finished nursing after forty-five minutes, but maybe she needs more. I don't want her to starve.	She's not starving. She just misses the company of your left boob, which is now her closest friend.
I should cherish every single second of a nursing session . . . so why do I often feel bored out of my mind?	Try this exercise: cherish (two minutes); read tabloid magazine (five minutes); cherish (two minutes); read tabloid magazine (five minutes). Repeat.
I shouldn't be introducing formula. What about my baby's IQ? His immune system? He should be getting breast milk exclusively—it's the best for him, right?	Formula is not your enemy. Indeed, it may become your best friend.

GUILT TRIP YOU PULL ON YOURSELF	REALITY
I shouldn't introduce the pacifier since it can lead to nipple confusion.	Are your nipples abnormally long, rounded, and attached to plastic holders? If so, you may need to worry (and not just because of the nipple confusion).
I shouldn't be sitting around all the time doing nothing while I nurse. I need to be productive!	Repeat this phrase in your mind until it becomes one of your most deeply held truths: "Watching Oprah is productive." "Watching Oprah is productive."
Why am I not producing more milk? I'm not providing for my baby!	Trust your boobs. They know way more about this than you do, and they're no doubt stepping up production even as you read this.
Yes, I may have a broken rib, but if I take the pain medication my doctor prescribed, my baby will become a drug addict.	If you got the green light from your doctor and pediatrician, step on the gas and merge onto Drug Highway as fast as you can.

YOU, the NON-MOM

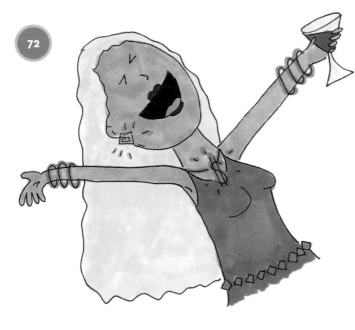

New motherhood wearing you down? Use your imagination to escape for a moment. Picture your glamorous life as a semiscandalous young socialite. You're dressed to the nines, speeding around in a head-turning car, and getting waved into all of the hip clubs. If only the paparazzi would leave you alone!

What would be the name of your socialite alter ego? Use this formula to find out.

**Your socialite name
=
Disney princess who
looks most like you
+
Ritziest suburb near
your hometown**

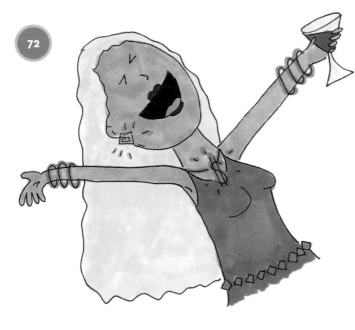

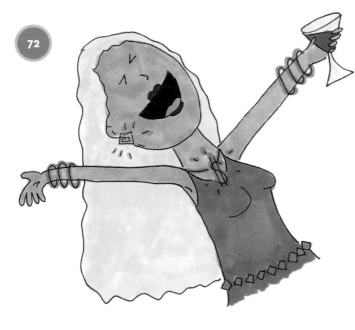

MATCH THE NUMBER TO THE STATEMENT

Numbers	Statement
10	Number of times in a day you think your baby wants a full meal of milk, only to find out she just wanted a quick snack.
100	Number of times you think, "I can't possibly do this!" during the first week.
At least 20	Number of times baby falls asleep at the boob during the first week.
Less than 1	Number of minutes a man could handle breast-feeding a child, if he had the anatomy to do so.
7	Number of minutes you have to yourself between feeding sessions.
126	Number of times you change breast pads in the first month.
4	Number of times a day you wonder how cave women survived without breast pumps, doctors, and parenting chat rooms.

DREAM ON

Do you have bizarre dreams now that you've entered the world of mommyhood? Here's what experts say your dreams—if you sleep long enough to have them—may symbolize:

SYMBOL	MEANING
Crying baby	You're deprived of attention and need nurturing
Baby shower	You're excited about a new start
Calling a babysitter	You need to work on your inner child
You wet the bed	Lack of control in your life
Blanket	Seeking shelter from something
Nursing	Nurturing a hidden aspect of yourself

SYMBOL	MEANING
Pacifier	Desire to escape from daily duties
Taking a pregnancy test	Entering into new phase of life
Baby carriage	A good friend pleasantly surprises you
Bathtubs	Need to escape everyday problems
Sleeping in your bed	Looking for security, peace
Pregnant belly	Need to express emotions
Empty bottle	You've exhausted yourself
Burping	Overcoming obstacles
Contraceptive	Not allowing your creativity to emerge

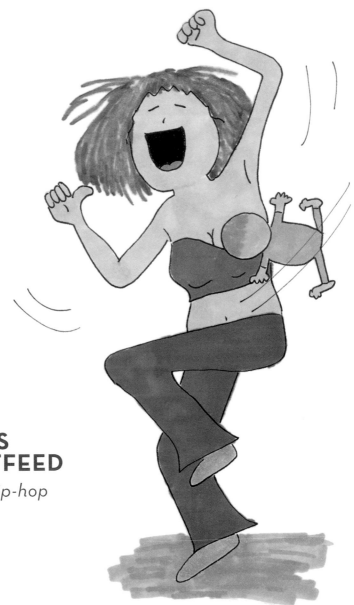

BAD TIMES to BREASTFEED

#5: During a hip-hop dance class

top ten inconvenient phobias
when you have a baby

1. Autodysomophobia—Fear of one that has a vile odor

2. Dishabiliophobia—Fear of undressing
in front of someone

3. Peladophobia—Fear of bald people

4. Pentheraphobia—Fear of mother-in-law

5. Scopophobia—Fear of being stared at

6. Proctophobia—Fear of rectums

7. Ponophobia—Fear of overworking

8. Emetophobia—Fear of vomiting

9. Maniaphobia—Fear of insanity

10. Pediophobia—Fear of children

THE RISE AND FALL
OF A-CUP BOOBS as told in theme songs

When you've collected a drawer full of gigundo nursing bras
Theme song: "Material Girl"

First few weeks after birth
Theme song: "You Shook Me All Night Long"

78

Engorgement Day
Theme song: "Pressure"

Pregnancy
Theme song: "We've Only Just Begun"

Pre-pregnancy
Theme song: "Tiny Bubbles"

Once you get the hang of nursing
Theme song: "What a Feeling"

First few months
Theme song: "Hopelessly Devoted to You"

When baby begins to bite
Theme song: "Cool It Now"

When baby decides to wean
Theme song: "Stay (Just a Little Bit Longer)"

Baby has weaned
Theme song: "Don't You Forget About Me," then "Margaritaville"

Your boobs shrink back to pre-pregnancy size or less
Theme song: "Dust in the Wind"

ALTERNATIVE USES for nursing pads

As breastfeeding winds down, you may find yourself with dozens of nursing pads that suddenly have no use. But wait! All is not lost. Try these innovative strategies to give your little buddies a second lease on life:

- Use them as coasters. You know how absorbent they are.
- Two words: toddler Frisbee
- Use them as oven pads (best to duct tape several together).
- You did need some more nonskid pads for your furniture, right?
- Spare tire covers for remote-controlled Jeep. Of course!
- Paint them with glow paint and tape to ceiling for homemade glow-in-the-dark solar system.
- Use them as elbow and knee pads—and a fashion statement too!
- Slide a metal rod through the center of ten pads and make your own abacus. (Note: This could be more trouble than it's worth.)
- Etch a little design in the center so they look like sand dollars. Place them tastefully around your home to create a beach motif.
- Fold them into cone shapes and use them as emergency drinking cups. (Best not to offer them to guests.)

BREASTFEEDING FIRSTS

You'll never forget . . .

- The first time baby looked up sweetly at your face while you were nursing her

- The first time baby pulled away from your breast and was startled by milk spraying in her face

- The first time you saw your breast milk when you pumped it out

- The first time you accidentally spilled the breast milk you just pumped, and began to panic

- The first time you forgot to wear a breastfeeding-friendly outfit

- The first time you leaked and realized you weren't wearing breast pads

- The first time you enjoyed a nice nursing session with baby, only to have baby spit-up all over your chest

LET IT GO

You know it's time to stop breastfeeding when your child:

- Text messages you to tell you he's hungry

- Mixes your milk with a shot of espresso

- Knows how to repair a broken pump

- Comes home from college needing more bags of frozen milk

- Can say "lactation" in two other languages

- Only wants to nurse during halftime so he won't miss any important plays of the game

- Is concerned about the fat content in your milk

- Uses the Boppy to also balance his sushi platter

This is too
difficult!

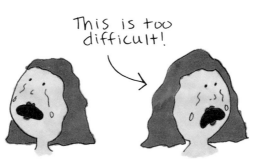

I don't want
it to be over!

What did
these huge
rocks do
with my
boobs?

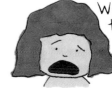

Oh no!
I see
the end
in sight.

Time to feed again...
Time to feed again...
Time to feed again...

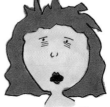

I
love
breastfeeding!

Hmm...this is
getting easier.

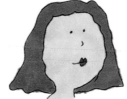

BREASTFEEDING CIRCLE OF LIFE

BOOB RETIREMENT PARTY

Your boobs have worked hard. Perhaps a nice retirement party is in order! Here's how to throw one.

1. Hang a colorful banner

2. Provide donuts, bagels, and other round food

3. Create a slideshow set to the tune "I've Had the Time of My Life"

4. Serve champagne (that you can drink without any guilt!)

5. Exchange stories and memories about your breastfeeding adventures

6. Invite your "coworkers" (i.e., lactation consultant, breast pump, and "how-to" book)

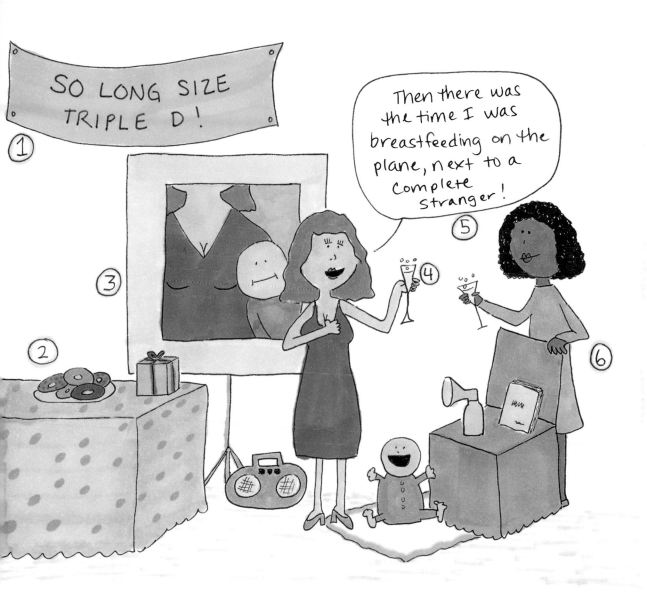

BOOBY STARS

Once nursing is over, what's next for your boobs? Perhaps a career in Hollywood? Just imagine if some of your favorite movies had a breastfeeding twist.

- -

"May the nursing pad be with you."
Pump Wars

"Here's looking at your hungry mouth, kid."
Casaboobca

"You can't *handle* the milk!"
A Few Good Boobs

"Life is like the first week of breastfeeding . . . you never know what you're gonna get."
Forrest Pump

"Frankly, pump, I don't give an ounce!"
Gone With the Milk

"I'll make him a milk he can't refuse."
The Godboober

"That's right, Ice Man: I *am* engorged."
Top Boob

"Show me the breast milk!"
Booby Maguire

"Boobs, I've got a feeling we're not in a B-cup anymore."
The Wizard of Breastfeeding

"Houston, we have a milk leak."
Aboobo 13

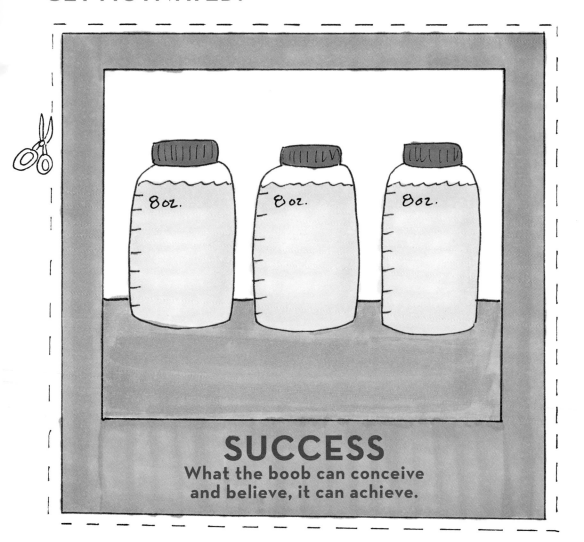

THANK YOU, BOOBS.
THANK YOU.

It's only polite to write a thank-you note when someone does something really special for you and your baby. Here's a note you can deliver to your boobs when the time is right.

Dear Boobs,

Where to begin? I don't think any of us knew what we were getting into, but look: We did it!

Your unwavering dedication to feeding the baby has been truly inspiring. Along the way, you've had ups and downs, and ups and downs . . . about every three to four hours, in fact.

Remember the time you couldn't even fit into one of my old T-shirts? Or when you started to leak and I had no nursing pads? Wow. We really had some crazy times, didn't we?

Things are changing now, though. Baby will grow, I will tend to baby, and you will try to cope with your shockingly diminished size. (We'll get one of those push-up bras . . . see if we can salvage some of your glory.)

At any rate, I want to thank you, Boobs. For providing food around the clock. For knowing what to do even when I didn't know. And for always being there for me and the baby. You made me proud.

You might feel slightly droopy now, but in my eyes you'll always be spectacular.

Sincerely,
Me